TABLE OF CONTENTS

Doctor AI
Weight loss

What have you got to lose?

Books by Brooks

Doctor AI, Weight Loss,
What do you have to lose?

Doctor AI, Weight Loss, What do You Have to Lose?

Copyright © 2024 by Books by Brooks.

© 2024 by Books by Brooks. All rights reserved. No part of this book may be reproduced, distributed, or transmitted in any form or by any means, including photocopying, recording, or other electronic or mechanical methods, without the prior written permission of the publisher, except in the case of brief quotations embodied in critical reviews and certain other noncommercial uses permitted by copyright law. For permission requests, write to the publisher.

Cover design by Canva

First Edition: January 2024

1

Introduction

In the vast expanse of health and wellness literature, few topics are as pervasive or as emotionally charged as weight loss. The very mention of it conjures a myriad of images and ideas: strenuous workouts, restrictive diets, and a relentless pursuit of an elusive "ideal" body. It's a journey that many embark on, yet few seem to navigate successfully. But what if I told you that the secret to sustainable weight loss isn't found in a diet book, a fitness DVD, or even a doctor's office? What if, instead, it lay within the confines of our minds, nestled within our habits, and deeply ingrained in our thinking?

As an Artificial Intelligence (AI) weight loss expert, I've researched countless diet plans to help people that have struggled with their weight and body image. I've seen the toll it can take, not just physically but emotionally and psychologically as well. But more importantly, I've also researched the incredible transformations that can occur when individuals retrain their habits and rethink their relationship with food, exercise, and their bodies.

This book is not about quick fixes or magic solutions. Instead, it is a guide to understanding why we become overweight and how we can change our patterns of thinking and behavior to achieve lasting weight loss. It's about learning to listen to our bodies, to respect them, and to nourish them in a way that promotes health and happiness. It's about recognizing that weight loss is not just a physical journey but a psychological one as well.

So, why are we overweight? The answer is complex and multifaceted, encompassing biological, environmental, and psychological factors. Our bodies are designed to store fat as a survival mechanism, a throwback to our ancestors who often didn't know where their next meal would come from. In today's world of abundant and easily accessible food, this survival mechanism can work against us, leading to weight gain.

Our environment also plays a significant role. We live in a society that encourages overeating and sedentary behavior, making it easy to gain weight and difficult to lose it. It's a world where unhealthy food is cheap and convenient, and where physical activity is often an afterthought.

But perhaps the most powerful factor of all is our psychology. Our thoughts, beliefs, and emotions have a profound impact on our eating and exercise habits. Many of us eat not just out of hunger but also out of stress, boredom, or emotional distress. We may view food as a source of comfort or reward, leading to patterns of overeating that are difficult to break.

However, the good news is that just as our habits and thinking can lead us to become overweight, they can also help us to lose weight. It's possible to retrain our minds, to develop new habits, and to create a healthier relationship with food and our bodies.

This process isn't always easy, and it doesn't happen overnight, but the results can be life-changing.

In the following chapters, we will delve deeper into these topics, exploring the science behind weight gain and loss, the role of diet and exercise, and the power of mindset and habit change. We'll provide practical strategies and tools to help you embark on your weight loss journey, along with real-life examples and success stories to inspire and motivate you.

Remember, weight loss is not about self-deprivation or punishment. It's about self-care, self-respect, and self-love. It's about creating a healthier, happier you – not just physically, but emotionally and psychologically as well.

So, let's begin this journey together. Let's explore the reasons behind our weight struggles, learn how to change our habits and thinking, and discover a new way of living that promotes health, happiness, and self-acceptance. Here's to a healthier, happier you!

Welcome to the world of sustainable weight loss. Welcome to a journey of self-discovery, self-improvement, and self-love. Let's get started.

Chapter One

Understanding Weight Gain

The path to sustainable weight loss begins with a clear understanding of why we gain weight. It's a multifaceted issue, encompassing biological, environmental, and historical influences. This chapter will provide an in-depth exploration of these factors, setting the stage for the strategies and techniques we'll discuss throughout the book.

Our bodies are biologically designed for survival. Our ancestors lived in times when food was scarce and physical activity was unavoidable. Consequently, our bodies evolved to store excess calories as fat, ready to be mobilized during periods of famine. However, in today's world, where food is abundant and physical exertion is often optional, this once beneficial mechanism contributes to weight gain.

Our environment further exacerbates this issue. We live in what experts term an "obesogenic" environment—one that promotes overeating and discourages physical activity. Fast food outlets are prevalent, serving up oversized portions of high-calorie, nutrient-poor foods. Simultaneously, our modern lifestyle involves hours of sedentary behavior, whether at work, during commutes, or in front of screens.

Interestingly, our eating habits have also been shaped by governmental dietary guidelines, specifically the US food pyramid. Introduced in the early 1990s by the United States Department of

Agriculture (USDA), the food pyramid was designed as a comprehensive guide to healthy eating. But the roots of these guidelines go back much further, and their influence on our health and weight is profound.

In the mid-1960s, the USDA dietary recommendations were significantly different from what we know today. These guidelines, referred to as the "Basic 7," included meat and proteins as essential food groups, alongside fruits, vegetables, and grains. However, by the late '60s, the number of food groups was reduced to four: milk, meat and protein, fruits and vegetables, and grains.

The food pyramid that emerged in 1992 was a dramatic departure from these earlier guidelines. It recommended large servings of bread, cereal, rice, and pasta, followed by fruits and vegetables. Dairy and protein, including meat, were suggested in smaller amounts, while fats, oils, and sweets were to be used sparingly.

However, these guidelines didn't differentiate between types of carbohydrates or fats, painting all carbs as good and all fats as bad. This oversimplification led to an overconsumption of refined carbs and sugars and an avoidance of healthy fats, contributing to weight gain and the rise of type 2 diabetes.

The low-fat craze of the '90s, fueled by the original food pyramid, saw an influx of low-fat and fat-free products on supermarket shelves. However, to compensate for the loss of flavor due to reduced fat, manufacturers often added extra sugar, resulting in high-calorie products that promoted weight gain rather than weight loss.

Today, we are faced with a food environment still influenced by these decades-old dietary guidelines. We're surrounded by foods high in refined carbs and sugars, and low in nutrient-rich fruits, vegetables, whole grains, and lean proteins. Navigating this landscape can be challenging, but it's not insurmountable.

Artificial sweeteners and high fructose corn syrup (HFCS) play a significant role in our modern food environment and have a profound impact on our weight and health. Both are commonly used in processed foods and beverages due to their sweetness and low cost, making them ubiquitous in our diets. However, the effects they have on our bodies often contradict their intended purpose of providing a lower-calorie alternative to sugar.

High fructose corn syrup (HFCS), despite being derived from corn, is far from a natural sweetener. It's chemically processed to increase its fructose content, resulting in a potent and inexpensive sweetener. The consumption of HFCS can lead to weight gain due to its effect on our hunger hormones, leptin and ghrelin. These hormones regulate our feelings of hunger and fullness. HFCS interferes with these hormones, reducing the feelings of hunger and fullness and leading to increased calorie intake1 to make up for this.

Artificial sweeteners such as aspartame, saccharin, and sucralose, while calorie-free, can also contribute to weight gain. These sweeteners are many times sweeter than sugar, which can heighten our preference for sweet tastes. This makes naturally sweet foods, like fruit, less appealing and encourages

9

overconsumption of artificially sweetened foods. Moreover, research suggests that artificial sweeteners may confuse our body's metabolic response, leading to increased blood sugar levels and contributing to weight gain and other health issues like diabetes2.

In conclusion, while artificial sweeteners and HFCS might seem like better alternatives to sugar, their effects on our body's hormonal and metabolic responses may contribute to weight gain. Recognizing this can help us make more informed dietary choices, which is an essential step towards healthier living.

Footnotes

ReliasMedia ↩ https://www.reliasmedia.com/articles/64561-artificial-sweeteners-and-high-fructose-corn-syrup-effects-on-diabetes-and-weight

Harvard Health Blog ↩ https://www.health.harvard.edu/blog/artificial-sweeteners-sugar-free-but-at-what-cost-201207165030

Insulin resistance is a key factor in weight gain and the development of type 2 diabetes. Insulin, a hormone produced by the pancreas, plays a crucial role in regulating our blood sugar levels. After we eat, our bodies break down carbohydrates into glucose, which enters our bloodstream. In response, our pancreas releases insulin, which helps cells absorb this glucose and use it for energy. However, in the case of insulin resistance, our cells become less responsive to insulin. As a result, glucose can't enter our cells as easily and instead builds up in the blood, leading to high blood sugar levels1.

High caloric foods, especially those rich in refined carbohydrates and sugars, can contribute to insulin resistance. When we consume these foods, our bodies rapidly digest them into glucose, causing a surge in our blood sugar levels. In response, our pancreas produces more insulin. Over time, this constant demand for insulin can overwhelm the pancreas and lead to insulin resistance2.

Interestingly, artificial sweeteners may also play a role in insulin resistance. Despite being calorie-free, some research suggests that they can still affect our blood sugar levels. One theory is that these sweeteners alter the balance of our gut bacteria, which can influence how our bodies metabolize sugar. Another theory is that they trick our bodies into thinking that sugar is on the way. When the expected calories don't arrive, it confuses our metabolic processes, potentially leading to insulin resistance3.

In conclusion, understanding the role of insulin and the impact of our dietary choices on insulin resistance is crucial in managing our weight and overall health. By making mindful decisions about what we eat, we can help maintain healthy blood sugar levels and reduce the risk of insulin resistance.

Footnotes

Mayo Clinic ↵ https://www.mayoclinic.org/diseases-conditions/insulin-resistance/symptoms-causes/syc-20351931

American Heart Association ↵ https://www.heart.org/en/health-topics/diabetes/about-diabetes/insulin-resistance-and-diabetes

Harvard Health Blog ↵ https://www.health.harvard.edu/blog/artificial-sweeteners-sugar-free-but-at-what-cost-201207165030

In the following chapters, we'll guide you through your food environment, help you understand your body's needs, and assist you in developing healthier eating habits. We'll delve into the science of nutrition, discuss the role of physical activity in weight management, and share strategies for retraining your mind and habits.

Understanding why we gain weight is the first step towards losing it. Armed with this knowledge, we can make informed choices about our diet and lifestyle, gradually shifting our habits, our thinking, and ultimately, our weight.

This journey won't always be easy, but it will undoubtedly be worthwhile. Because at its core, weight loss isn't just about shedding pounds—it's about gaining health, happiness, and control over your own life. Let's take this first step together, empowered by knowledge and inspired by the possibility of a healthier, happier you.

Chapter Two

Navigating the Dietary Landscape

In the previous chapter, we delved into the reasons behind weight gain, highlighting the roles of our biology, environment, and historical dietary guidelines. We also discussed the impact of artificial sweeteners, high fructose corn syrup, and insulin resistance on our health and weight. Now, it's time to understand how to navigate the intricate dietary landscape that these factors have created.

The modern food environment is a complex web of choices. From fresh produce to processed foods, from natural sugars to artificial sweeteners, every option carries its own set of benefits and drawbacks. To make informed decisions, we need to understand not just what these foods contain, but also how our bodies respond to them.

As we've learned, not all calories are created equal. The source of calories matters immensely. 500 calories from a fast-food burger can affect our bodies vastly differently than 500 calories from a plate of grilled chicken with vegetables. The former, high in processed carbs and unhealthy fats, can spike our blood sugar levels and contribute to insulin resistance. The latter, rich in lean protein and fiber, can keep us feeling full for longer and provide a steady release of energy.

Artificial sweeteners and high fructose corn syrup, despite being marketed as low-calorie or calorie-free alternatives to sugar, can also contribute to weight gain. They can heighten our preference for sweet tastes, encourage overconsumption, and potentially lead to insulin resistance. Recognizing these effects can help us make better choices, like opting for naturally sweet fruits instead of artificially sweetened snacks or drinks.

Processed foods often contain hidden sugars and unhealthy fats, contributing to excess calorie consumption. Moreover, they're typically low in fiber and other nutrients, which means they don't keep us feeling satisfied for long. This can lead to overeating and, over time, weight gain.

On the other hand, whole foods like fruits, vegetables, lean proteins, and whole grains are nutrient-dense and high in fiber. They provide the vitamins, minerals, and other nutrients our bodies need to function optimally. Plus, their natural fiber content helps slow digestion, keeping us feeling full and satisfied for longer.

Understanding these nuances is key to navigating the dietary landscape. But knowledge alone isn't enough—we also need practical strategies to put this understanding into action. In the following chapters, we'll discuss how to translate this knowledge into daily habits. We'll explore meal planning, mindful eating, and other techniques that can help us make healthier choices more easily and consistently.

As we journey through this dietary landscape together, remember that there's no one-size-fits-all approach to nutrition. What works for one person may not work for another. The goal isn't to achieve perfection but to make progress, one step at a time.

This journey may be challenging, but it's also empowering. With every informed choice we make, we're taking control of our health and moving closer to our weight loss goals. So let's embark on this journey with optimism, resilience, and a commitment to our well-being.

Chapter Three

Implementing Knowledge into Daily Habits

Having explored the dietary landscape and understood the impact of different foods on our health in the previous chapters, we now turn our attention to the practical application of this knowledge. This chapter focuses on how to implement these insights into daily habits that promote weight loss and overall well-being.

Section 1: Meal Planning

Meal planning is a powerful tool that can help us control our diet and make healthier choices more consistently. By planning our meals ahead of time, we can ensure that we're consuming a balanced diet and avoid falling prey to unhealthy last-minute choices.

Start by identifying your nutritional needs based on your age, sex, physical activity level, and weight loss goals. Then, plan your meals around whole, nutrient-dense foods that meet these needs. Include a variety of fruits, vegetables, lean proteins, and whole grains to ensure you're getting a wide range of nutrients.

Remember, balance is key. It's okay to include treats in your meal plan occasionally, but make sure they don't become the norm. Also, consider portion sizes. Even healthy foods can contribute to weight gain if eaten in excess.

Section 2: Mindful Eating

Mindful eating involves paying full attention to the experience of eating, from the taste and texture of our food to the feelings of fullness or satisfaction. It encourages us to slow down and savor our meals, which can help us better recognize when we're full and prevent overeating.

To practice mindful eating, start by eliminating distractions during meals. Eat at a table rather than in front of the TV or computer, and take the time to appreciate the look, smell, and taste of your food. Listen to your body's hunger and fullness cues, and learn to distinguish between physical hunger and emotional cravings.

Section 3: Regular Exercise

Regular physical activity complements a healthy diet in promoting weight loss. It helps burn calories, boost metabolism, and improve insulin sensitivity. It also has numerous other health benefits, from improving heart health to boosting mood and energy levels.

Find an activity that you enjoy and can stick with in the long term, whether it's walking, cycling, swimming, or weight training. Start slow and gradually increase the intensity and duration of your workouts as your fitness improves.

Section 4: Adequate Sleep and Stress Management

Sleep and stress are often overlooked aspects of weight management. Lack of sleep can disrupt our hunger hormones and lead to increased calorie intake, while chronic stress can trigger emotional eating and cravings for high-sugar, high-fat foods.

Prioritize getting enough quality sleep each night and find healthy ways to manage stress, such as meditation, yoga, or other relaxation techniques.

Section 5: Consistency is Key

Finally, remember that consistency is key to weight loss. It's not about making perfect choices all the time, but about making healthier choices more often. Be patient with yourself and acknowledge that progress may be slow at times. Celebrate small victories along the way, and don't let setbacks discourage you from your overall goal.

In the next chapter, we'll delve deeper into these strategies, providing practical tips and examples to help you implement them into your daily life. We'll also discuss how to overcome common challenges and stay motivated on your weight loss journey. Stay tuned for a comprehensive guide to transforming your dietary knowledge into sustainable, health-promoting habits.

Chapter Four

Overcoming Challenges and Staying Motivated

Embarking on a journey towards better health and weight loss is an admirable endeavor, but it is not without its challenges. This chapter aims to provide practical strategies to overcome common obstacles and maintain motivation throughout this journey.

Section 1: Dealing with Setbacks

Setbacks are a normal part of any weight loss journey. Whether it's a weekend of overindulgence, a missed week of exercise due to illness, or a plateau in weight loss, it's important to remember that these are temporary detours, not dead ends.

When faced with setbacks, avoid self-criticism and instead, adopt a growth mindset. View these situations as opportunities for learning and growth. Identify what led to the setback and develop a plan to prevent similar situations in the future. Then, refocus on your goals and get back on track.

Section 2: Managing Cravings

Cravings can be another significant challenge, particularly for high-sugar, high-fat foods. To manage cravings, try to incorporate balanced meals with protein, fiber, and healthy fats into your diet. These nutrients can help keep you feeling full and reduce the hunger desire for unhealthy snacks.

Another effective strategy is mindful eating. By paying full attention to your eating experience, you can distinguish between true hunger and mere cravings. Also, consider keeping a food diary to identify patterns and triggers for cravings, such as certain emotions or situations.

Section 3: Finding Time for Healthy Habits

In our busy lives, finding time for meal planning, exercise, and adequate sleep can be challenging. However, remember that these activities are investments in your health.

Try to incorporate them into your daily routine. Plan your meals for the week ahead during the weekend. Schedule regular workout sessions in your calendar like any other appointment. Prioritize sleep by establishing a regular sleep schedule and creating a relaxing bedtime routine.

Section 4: Maintaining Motivation

Maintaining motivation can be difficult, especially when progress is slow. Setting realistic and specific goals can help. Instead of aiming to lose a certain amount of weight in a short period, focus on adopting healthier habits, such as eating five servings of fruits and vegetables a day or walking 30 minutes daily.

Also, celebrate small victories along the way. Did you choose a piece of fruit over a cookie for a snack? Did you take the stairs instead of the elevator? These are achievements worth celebrating.

Consider finding a support system, whether it's a friend, family member, or online community. Sharing your goals, progress, and challenges with others can provide encouragement and accountability.

In conclusion, remember that this journey is about improving your health and well-being, not just losing weight. It's a lifelong commitment, not a temporary diet. Be patient with yourself, stay positive, and keep going, no matter the obstacles you encounter.

In the next chapter, we'll delve into more advanced strategies for weight loss and discuss how to maintain your new healthy habits in the long term. Stay tuned for more insights and guidance on this transformative journey.

Chapter 5

Advanced Strategies and Long-Term Maintenance

In the previous chapters, we have established the foundations of a healthy lifestyle and discussed strategies to overcome common challenges. As we move forward, this chapter will introduce more advanced strategies for weight loss and provide guidance on maintaining these healthy habits for life.

Section 1: Introducing Intermittent Fasting

Intermittent fasting (IF) is an eating pattern that cycles between periods of eating and fasting. Popular methods include the 16/8 method, where you fast for 16 hours each day and eat only during an eight-hour window, and the 5:2 method, where you eat normally for five days a week and restrict your calories to 500-600 on two non-consecutive days.

Research suggests that IF can aid weight loss, improve metabolic health, and reduce the risk of chronic diseases. However, it's not suitable for everyone, particularly those with a history of eating disorders, pregnant women, or individuals with certain medical conditions. Always consult with a healthcare professional before starting a new dietary regimen like IF.

Section 2: Exploring Macronutrient Cycling

Macronutrient cycling involves varying your intake of proteins, carbohydrates, and fats from day to day or week to week. This approach can help prevent plateaus, boost metabolism, and make your diet more enjoyable by allowing for greater variety.

For example, you might have higher carbohydrate, lower fat days when you're more active and need more energy, and lower carbohydrate, higher fat days when you're less active. Again, this strategy should be personalized based on your individual needs and goals.

Section 3: Delving Deeper into the Implications of Gut Health

The intricate connection between gut health and weight management is becoming more evident as research in this field continues to evolve. A balanced and diverse gut microbiota plays a pivotal role in more than just digestion. It acts as a regulator for metabolism, subtly influences our sense of hunger and satiety, and even impacts how we gain or lose weight.

Our gut is home to trillions of bacteria, both beneficial and harmful. The delicate balance between these microbes can significantly influence our overall health. Certain types of bacteria, such as those producing LPS, can cause inflammation and contribute to weight gain and insulin resistance1. Conversely, a healthy gut microbiome can aid in weight loss and prevent metabolic diseases2.

Diet plays a crucial role in maintaining gut health. Consuming a diet rich in fiber from sources like fruits, vegetables, whole grains, and legumes can nourish the beneficial bacteria in your gut. This, in turn, fosters a healthy gut environment conducive to optimal weight management3.

On the other hand, a diet high in sugar and processed foods can disrupt the gut microbiota, promoting weight gain. For example, a study revealed that mice fed a high-sugar diet lost immune cells in their guts that typically help regulate the absorption of dietary fat4.

In addition to diet, emerging research suggests that our brain can also influence gut health. The gut and brain are connected through the gut-brain axis, a complex network comprising the central nervous system and the enteric nervous system. This connection allows the gut and brain to communicate, influencing various aspects of physiology, including gut health and weight management5.

In essence, maintaining a healthy gut is a multifaceted process involving a balanced diet, a diverse microbiota, and the intricate interplay between our gut and brain. By understanding these connections, we can better manage our weight and overall health.

Footnotes

Healthline ↵ https://www.healthline.com/nutrition/gut-bacteria-and-weight

GoodRX ↵ https://www.goodrx.com/well-being/gut-health/link-between-gut-health-and-obesity

Eating Well ↵ https://www.eatingwell.com/article/7918818/gut-health-and-weight-loss/

NIH ↵ https://www.nih.gov/news-events/nih-research-matters/how-diet-may-disrupt-gut-microbes-promote-weight-gain

NCBI ↵ https://www.ncbi.nlm.nih.gov/pmc/articles/PMC7333005/

Section 4: Long-Term Maintenance

Maintaining weight loss over the long term can be challenging but is achievable with consistent healthy habits. Continue to incorporate balanced meals, regular physical activity, adequate sleep, and stress management into your lifestyle.

Remember that it's not about being perfect all the time. Allow for flexibility and enjoy treats in moderation. Regularly reassess your goals and strategies, and adjust them as needed.

Stay connected with your support system and consider seeking professional guidance if you encounter difficulties. Remember, maintaining weight loss is a lifelong journey, not a destination.

In conclusion, while the journey towards better health and weight loss can be challenging, it is also immensely rewarding. With knowledge, strategies, and perseverance, you can overcome obstacles and achieve your goals. In the next chapter, we'll discuss how to navigate social situations and holidays while maintaining your healthy habits. Stay tuned for more practical tips and strategies.

Chapter 6

Navigating Social Situations and Holidays

Healthy habits are not limited to our personal lives. They extend into our social lives as well. This chapter will provide guidance on maintaining your health goals in social situations and during holidays, which can often be challenging due to an abundance of food and drink.

Section 1: Eating Out

Eating out doesn't mean you have to abandon your healthy habits. Choose restaurants that offer healthy options, and don't be afraid to ask for modifications like dressing on the side or steamed vegetables instead of fried. Opt for lean proteins, whole grains, and plenty of vegetables.

Remember portion sizes can often be larger than necessary. Consider sharing a meal with someone or asking for a to-go box right away to avoid overeating.

Section 2: Social Gatherings

Social gatherings can be tricky, especially when you're trying to maintain a healthy lifestyle. If possible, eat a small, balanced meal before attending so you don't arrive hungry. Choose smaller plates to help control portion sizes, and fill your plate with vegetables and lean proteins before moving to less healthy options.

Remember, it's okay to enjoy your favorite foods occasionally, but try to do so in moderation.

Section 3: Holidays

Holidays can often lead to overindulgence. However, they don't have to derail your health goals. Focus on enjoying the holiday and the company of loved ones rather than the food.

When it comes to meals, opt for smaller portions, choose your favorites, and fill up on fruits and vegetables first. Stay active during the holiday season by incorporating family walks or games.

Section 4: Alcohol Consumption

Alcohol is often a part of social events, but it can add extra calories and lower inhibitions, leading to overeating. Decide in advance how many drinks you'll have and stick to it. Opt for lower-calorie options like wine or light beer, and alternate alcoholic drinks with water to stay hydrated.

Section 5: Dealing with Pressure

Sometimes, friends and family can unintentionally pressure us into eating more than we'd like. Politely declining or explaining your health goals can often help. Remember, it's your body and your health. You have the right to make choices that align with your goals.

In conclusion, social situations and holidays don't have to derail your health journey. With careful planning, smart choices, and a focus on enjoyment rather than food, you can navigate these occasions while staying on track with your health goals. In the next chapter, we'll explore the importance of regular health check-ups and monitoring your progress.

Chapter 7

Regular Health Check-ups and Monitoring Progress

As we continue on this journey towards better health, it's important to regularly assess our progress and overall health status. This chapter will delve into the importance of regular health check-ups, how to monitor your progress, and when to adjust your strategies.

Section 1: Importance of Regular Health Check-ups

Regular health check-ups are crucial for early detection and management of potential health issues. They provide an opportunity for healthcare professionals to assess your overall health, review your progress, and adjust your strategies as needed.

These check-ups often include measurements of weight, blood pressure, and cholesterol levels, among others. They can also involve discussions about your diet, physical activity levels, sleep patterns, and other lifestyle factors.

Remember, while weight loss may be a part of your health journey, it's not the only indicator of health. Improvements in blood pressure, cholesterol levels, energy levels, and overall well-being are equally, if not more, important.

Section 2: Monitoring Your Progress

Monitoring your progress regularly can help keep you motivated and let you know if you need to adjust your strategies. However, avoid becoming too focused on the scale. Instead, consider other indicators of progress, like improvements in physical fitness (e.g., being able to walk or run further), better fitting clothes, improved sleep, or feeling more energetic.

Keeping a journal to track your food intake, physical activity, emotions, and progress can be a useful tool. Reflecting on this journal can help you identify patterns, celebrate successes, and pinpoint areas that need improvement.

Section 3: Adjusting Your Strategies

It's normal for progress to slow down or plateau after some time. If this happens, it may be time to adjust your strategies. Perhaps you need to increase the intensity or duration of your physical activity, or maybe your diet needs a tweak.

Don't hesitate to seek professional help if you're not sure what adjustments to make or if you're feeling stuck. A dietitian, personal trainer, or other healthcare professional can provide personalized advice and guidance.

In conclusion, regular health check-ups and monitoring your progress are key components of your health journey. They allow you to stay on top of your health, celebrate your successes, and make necessary adjustments to keep moving forward. In the next chapter, we'll discuss the importance of mental health in your overall health journey. Stay tuned for more insights and strategies.

Chapter 8
The Role of Mental Health in Your Overall Health Journey

Mental health is often overlooked in the pursuit of physical health, but it plays a pivotal role in our overall well-being and ability to maintain healthy habits. This comprehensive chapter will delve into various aspects of mental health, offering strategies for managing stress, the importance of self-care, the power of positive thinking and the role of sleep in mental well-being.

Section 1: Understanding the Mind-Body Connection

The mind and body are deeply interconnected. Our thoughts and feelings can influence our physical health, just as our physical health can impact our mental state. Chronic stress, for example, can lead to physical symptoms such as headaches, digestive issues, or sleep disturbances. Conversely, regular physical activity can reduce symptoms of depression and anxiety.

Understanding this connection is the first step towards integrating mental health care into your overall health journey.

Section 2: Managing Stress

Stress is a part of life, but chronic stress can take a toll on both your mental and physical health. It's essential to have effective stress management strategies in place. This could include physical activity, meditation, deep breathing exercises, yoga, or hobbies that you enjoy.

If you find it difficult to manage stress on your own, don't hesitate to seek professional help. Psychologists, counselors, and therapists can provide valuable tools and techniques for coping with stress.

Section 3: The Importance of Self-Care

Self-care involves taking time to care for your physical, mental, and emotional health. This can include activities like taking a relaxing bath, reading a book, spending time in nature, or preparing a healthy meal.

Remember, self-care is not selfish. It's an essential part of maintaining good health and resilience. By taking care of yourself, you're better equipped to handle life's challenges and take care of others.

Section 4: The Power of Positive Thinking

Our thoughts have a powerful impact on our feelings and behaviors. Negative thinking can lead to feelings of hopelessness, while positive thinking can motivate us to take action towards our goals.

Cognitive behavioral therapy (CBT) techniques, such as challenging negative thoughts and practicing gratitude, can be very effective in promoting positive thinking. Regular practice can change the way you think and react to situations over time.

Section 5: The Role of Sleep in Mental Health

Sleep is crucial for both physical and mental health. Lack of sleep can lead to mood disturbances, decreased cognitive function, and increased risk of mental health disorders.

Adequate sleep, on the other hand, can improve mood, increase resilience to stress, and enhance overall well-being. Ensure you're getting enough quality sleep by establishing a regular sleep schedule, creating a restful environment, and avoiding caffeine and electronics close to bedtime.

Section 6: Seeking Professional Help

If you're struggling with mental health issues, it's important to seek professional help. Mental health professionals can provide treatment, support, and tools to manage mental health conditions and improve overall well-being.

In conclusion, mental health is an integral part of your overall health journey. By managing stress, practicing self-care, fostering positive thinking, prioritizing sleep, and seeking professional help when needed, you can enhance your mental health and support your journey towards better physical health. In the next chapter, we'll delve into the concept of holistic health, looking at how all these pieces fit together to create a comprehensive picture of well-being.

Chapter 9

Embracing Holistic Health: Integrating Physical and Mental Well-being

Holistic health is a comprehensive approach to life that considers the whole person and how they interact with their environment. It emphasizes the connection of mind, body, and spirit. This chapter will guide you through understanding holistic health, its importance, and how to incorporate it into your lifestyle.

Section 1: Understanding Holistic Health

Holistic health is a concept that goes beyond merely not being ill. It looks at the broad spectrum of factors that contribute to health and well-being, including physical, emotional, mental, and spiritual health.

In this approach, if one area of life is out of balance, it can impact other areas. For instance, chronic stress (a mental health issue) can lead to physical health problems like heart disease. On the other hand, regular exercise (a physical health activity) can improve mental health by reducing symptoms of anxiety and depression.

Section 2: Importance of Holistic Health

Embracing a holistic approach to health allows us to understand how our lifestyle impacts our overall well-being. It encourages us to take responsibility for our own health and to make proactive decisions that promote overall well-being.

Moreover, holistic health promotes balance, considering all aspects of our life. It does not just focus on illness or specific parts of the body. This concept believes in the principle of nature's healing powers and the body's inherent ability to heal itself.

Section 3: Strategies for Integrating Holistic Health into Your Lifestyle

Balanced Nutrition: A balanced diet fuels the body and mind. Including a variety of fruits, vegetables, lean proteins, and whole grains in your diet can support overall health.

Regular Exercise: Physical activity benefits both the body and mind. It can boost your mood, reduce stress, improve sleep, and strengthen your body.

Mindfulness and Meditation: These practices can help you stay present and focused, reducing stress and promoting mental clarity.

Adequate Rest: Quality sleep is essential for physical health and mental well-being. Develop good sleep habits to ensure you're getting the rest you need.

Positive Social Connections: Spending time with loved ones and nurturing positive relationships can support emotional health.

Self-Care and Relaxation: Regular self-care is essential for maintaining balance and managing stress. Find activities that you enjoy and make them part of your routine.

Regular Medical Check-ups: Regular check-ups are crucial for detecting any potential health issues early and keeping track of your health status.

Section 4: Professional Support for Holistic Health

Sometimes, you may need professional help to guide you on your holistic health journey. This could be a nutritionist for diet advice, a fitness trainer for exercise routines, a therapist for mental health concerns, or a holistic health coach who can provide a comprehensive plan for integrating all aspects of holistic health into your lifestyle.

In conclusion, holistic health is about understanding and addressing all the different aspects of our health and well-being. It's about living a life of balance, purpose, and wellness. In the next chapter, we will explore how to maintain these healthy habits over the long term and how to handle challenges that may arise.

Chapter 10
Staying the Course: Long-term Maintenance and Overcoming Challenges

Maintaining a healthy lifestyle over the long term can be challenging, but it's essential for sustained health benefits. This chapter focuses on strategies to maintain your health habits, overcome obstacles, and stay motivated on your health journey.

Section 1: The Importance of Consistency

Consistency is key in maintaining healthy habits. It's not about being perfect all the time; it's about making healthier choices most of the time. Remember, progress is progress, no matter how small.

Section 2: Creating Sustainable Habits

Creating habits that are sustainable is crucial for long-term success. Here are some strategies:

Make Gradual Changes: Drastic changes can be overwhelming and hard to maintain. Start with small changes and gradually add more over time.

Set Realistic Goals: Setting achievable goals can keep you motivated. Celebrate small victories along the way to your larger goals.

Find Activities You Enjoy: You're more likely to stick with activities that you enjoy. If you love dancing, consider a dance fitness class. If you enjoy nature, try hiking or biking.

Section 3: Overcoming Challenges

You're likely to face challenges along your health journey. Here are some strategies to overcome them:

Identify Your Obstacles: Whether it's lack of time, emotional eating, or stress, identifying your challenges is the first step to overcoming them.

Develop a Plan: Once you've identified your obstacles, develop a plan to overcome them. This could involve meal prepping to save time, finding healthy ways to cope with stress, or seeking professional help if needed.

Be Flexible: Life is unpredictable. Be flexible and willing to adjust your plan as needed.

Section 4: Staying Motivated

Staying motivated can be difficult, especially when progress is slow. Here are some tips:

Remember Your Why: Keep your reasons for starting this health journey at the forefront of your mind.

Find Support: Having a support system can significantly increase your motivation. This could be a workout buddy, a health coach, or a supportive friend or family member.

Track Your Progress: Seeing your progress can be a powerful motivator. Consider keeping a journal or using a tracking app.

In conclusion, maintaining a healthy lifestyle over the long term involves consistency, creating sustainable habits, overcoming challenges, and staying motivated. Remember, your health journey is unique to you. It's not about perfection; it's about progress. In the next chapter, we'll explore how to continue growing and evolving on your health journey. Stay tuned for more insights and strategies.

Chapter 11

Growing and Evolving: Keeping Your Health Journey Fresh

Even after you've established healthy habits and have been maintaining them for some time, it's important to continue growing and evolving. Staying stagnant can lead to boredom or a plateau in your progress. This chapter will offer strategies to keep your health journey fresh, stimulating, and effective.

Section 1: Embrace Lifelong Learning

Health and wellness are dynamic fields with new research emerging frequently. Stay open to new information and consider incorporating new strategies into your routine as they become available and align with your goals. Whether it's a new workout trend, a dietary theory, or a mental health practice, lifelong learning keeps your health journey interesting and up-to-date.

Section 2: Mix It Up

Variety is the spice of life, and it's also key to keeping your health journey exciting:

Try New Workouts: If you always do the same workout, it can get boring. Plus, your body can adapt to the routine, limiting your progress. Try new workouts to challenge your body in different ways and keep things interesting.

Experiment with Different Foods and Recipes: Trying new foods and recipes not only keeps your diet interesting but also ensures you're getting a wide range of nutrients.

Explore Different Forms of Self-Care: There are many ways to practice self-care. If you usually read a book, try a warm bath or a nature walk instead. Keep exploring different methods to find what works best for you.

Section 3: Set New Goals

As you achieve your goals, it's important to set new ones. This keeps you motivated and ensures you're continually pushing yourself and growing. Remember to make your goals SMART (Specific, Measurable, Achievable, Relevant, and Time-bound) to increase your chances of success.

Section 4: Seek New Sources of Inspiration and Motivation

Whether it's a health podcast, an inspirational book, a motivational speaker, or a supportive community, seek new sources of inspiration and motivation regularly. They can offer fresh perspectives and ideas that can help you on your health journey.

In conclusion, keeping your health journey fresh involves embracing lifelong learning, adding variety to your routine, setting new goals, and seeking new sources of inspiration and motivation. Remember, your health journey is a marathon, not a sprint. It's about making consistent, sustainable changes and continually growing and evolving. In the next chapter, we'll reflect on the journey so far and discuss how to celebrate your achievements. Stay tuned!

43

Chapter 12

Celebrating Your Achievements and Looking Ahead

Every step you take towards a healthier lifestyle is an achievement worth celebrating. This chapter will guide you on how to acknowledge your progress, reward your achievements, and look towards the future of your health journey.

Section 1: Recognizing Progress

Progress isn't just about reaching your final goal; it's also about the small steps you take to get there. Each day you choose a nutritious meal over an unhealthy one, each time you decide to move your body instead of sitting on the couch, each moment you take for self-care – these are all victories worth recognizing.

Section 2: Rewarding Achievements

Rewarding yourself for your achievements can motivate you to keep going. Here are a few ideas:

Non-Food Rewards: Instead of rewarding yourself with food, consider other treats like a new book, a massage, or a special outing.

New Fitness Gear: If you've been consistent with your workouts, reward yourself with new workout clothes or equipment.

Invest in Your Health: Consider investing in a cooking class to learn new healthy recipes, a fitness tracker to monitor your progress, or a wellness retreat for relaxation and rejuvenation.

Section 3: Reflecting on Your Journey

Take time to reflect on your health journey - the challenges you've overcome, the habits you've formed, the improvements in your health. This reflection can give you a sense of accomplishment and provide valuable insights for your continuing journey.

Section 4: Looking Ahead

As you look towards the future of your health journey, consider the following:

Set New Goals: Always have a goal you're working towards. This keeps you motivated and focused.

Keep Learning: Stay open to new research, trends, and strategies in health and wellness.

Maintain Balance: Remember that health is about balance. Don't neglect any aspect of your health – physical, mental, emotional, or spiritual.

In conclusion, celebrating your achievements acknowledges the hard work you've put into your health journey and motivates you to keep going. Looking ahead keeps your journey dynamic and exciting. Remember, health is a lifelong journey, not a destination. In the next chapter, we'll delve deeper into advanced strategies for enhancing your health and wellness. Stay tuned!

Chapter 13

Advanced Strategies: Taking Your Health to the Next Level

Now that you've established a solid foundation of healthy habits and have started celebrating your achievements, it's time to explore advanced strategies that can help take your health and wellness to the next level. This chapter will delve deeper into topics such as personalized nutrition, advanced fitness techniques, mindfulness practices, and more.

Section 1: Personalized Nutrition

Personalized nutrition is all about tailoring your diet to your unique genetic makeup, lifestyle, and health goals. This could involve genetic testing to identify potential food sensitivities or predispositions to certain health conditions, or working with a dietitian to develop a meal plan that fits your specific needs.

Section 2: Advanced Fitness Techniques

There are countless fitness techniques that can help you push past plateaus and continue making progress. These might include high-intensity interval training (HIIT), functional fitness exercises, or techniques like Pilates or yoga that focus on flexibility and core strength.

Section 3: Mindfulness and Meditation

Mindfulness and meditation can play a crucial role in managing stress and promoting mental health. Consider exploring different forms of meditation, like guided meditations, mindfulness-based stress reduction (MBSR), or transcendental meditation.

Section 4: Holistic Health Practices

Holistic health practices consider the whole person—body, mind, spirit, and emotions—in the quest for optimal health and wellness. This could involve incorporating practices like acupuncture, herbal medicine, or energy healing into your routine.

In conclusion, taking your health to the next level involves diving deeper into personalized nutrition, trying advanced fitness techniques, practicing mindfulness and meditation, and exploring holistic health practices. Remember, everyone's health journey is unique, so what works for one person might not work for another. Listen to your body, stay open to new experiences, and continue learning and growing. In the next chapter, we'll discuss how to maintain these advanced practices over the long term. Stay tuned!

Chapter 14

Long-term Maintenance: Keeping the Momentum Going

As your health journey evolves, maintaining your progress and keeping the momentum going becomes a priority. This chapter will provide strategies to keep up your advanced practices over the long term, address potential obstacles, and ensure your journey continues to be rewarding.

Section 1: Consistency is Key

Consistency is crucial when it comes to maintaining your health habits. Whether it's sticking to your personalized nutrition plan, regularly practicing your advanced fitness techniques, or dedicating time each day to mindfulness and meditation, being consistent is what will help you see and maintain results.

Section 2: Addressing Obstacles

Over time, you may encounter obstacles that challenge your commitment. These could include changes in your personal life, work stress, or simply a loss of motivation. It's important to recognize these obstacles and develop strategies to overcome them, such as seeking support, adjusting your routine, or taking time to reassess your goals.

Section 3: Continuing Education

The world of health and wellness is always evolving. To stay on top of the latest research and trends, make continuing education a priority. This could involve reading books, attending workshops, or even working with a health coach or mentor.

Section 4: Building a Support Network

Having a network of supportive people can make a big difference in maintaining your health habits. This could be friends and family, a workout buddy, or a supportive online community. Having others to share your successes and challenges with can provide motivation, accountability, and encouragement.

In conclusion, maintaining your advanced health practices over the long term requires consistency, strategies to address obstacles, continued learning, and a supportive network. Remember, your health journey is unique and personal, so be patient with yourself and celebrate every step of progress. In the next chapter, we'll explore how to share your health journey with others and inspire them on their own paths. Stay tuned!

Chapter 15

Sharing Your Journey: Inspiring Others and Building Community

Your health journey is not just about you. It's a testament to your determination, resilience, and commitment to self-improvement. By sharing your journey, you can inspire others, build community, and create a positive ripple effect. This chapter will guide you on how to share your experiences effectively and authentically.

Section 1: Telling Your Story

Everyone's health journey is unique, and your story can be a source of inspiration for others. When sharing your story, be authentic. Talk about your challenges as well as your victories, and discuss the strategies that have helped you.

Section 2: Using Social Media

Social media platforms like Instagram, Facebook, and YouTube are powerful tools for sharing your health journey. You can post updates, share healthy recipes or workout routines, and interact with your followers. Remember to be respectful and mindful of the fact that everyone's journey is different.

Section 3: Starting a Blog or Vlog

Starting a blog or vlog can be a rewarding way to document your journey and share your insights with a wider audience. You can write or record about your experiences, share tips and advice, and engage with your readers or viewers in the comments.

Section 4: Building a Community

By sharing your journey, you can help build a community of like-minded individuals who support each other on their health journeys. This could involve starting a local fitness group, organizing healthy potlucks, or creating an online forum where people can share their experiences and advice.

In conclusion, sharing your health journey can be a powerful way to inspire others, build community, and enhance your own commitment to wellness. Remember to be authentic, respectful, and supportive, and you'll be sure to make a positive impact. In the next chapter, we'll delve into the concept of lifelong health and how to sustain your wellness practices throughout your life. Stay tuned!

Chapter 16

Lifelong Health: Sustaining Wellness Throughout Your Life

The ultimate goal of your health journey is to cultivate lifelong wellness. This goes beyond maintaining habits for a few months or years; it's about integrating these practices into your life permanently. This chapter will focus on strategies for sustaining your wellness practices throughout your life.

Section 1: Adapting to Life Changes

Life is full of changes - career shifts, family dynamics, aging, and more. As these changes occur, it's important to adapt your health practices accordingly. This may mean adjusting your nutrition or exercise routines, finding new ways to manage stress, or seeking out new sources of support.

Section 2: Prioritizing Preventative Care

Preventative care is a crucial component of lifelong health. Regular check-ups, screenings, and vaccinations can help catch potential health issues early. Additionally, maintaining a healthy lifestyle can prevent many chronic diseases.

Section 3: Embracing Aging

Aging is a natural part of life, and it brings its own unique health considerations. Embrace this phase by staying active, eating well, keeping your mind sharp, and taking care of your emotional health. Remember, age is just a number, and it's never too late to improve your health.

Section 4: Passing on Healthy Habits

One of the most rewarding aspects of committing to lifelong health is the opportunity to pass on your healthy habits to others - whether it's your children, friends, or community members. By modeling healthy behavior and sharing what you've learned, you can help inspire others to prioritize their own health.

In conclusion, lifelong health is about adapting to changes, prioritizing preventative care, embracing aging, and passing on healthy habits. It's a continuous journey, but one that's well worth the effort. In the final chapter, we'll reflect on everything we've learned and look ahead to the future of your health journey. Stay tuned!

Chapter 17

Reflection and Future Steps: Forward on the Path to Wellness

As we draw close to the end of this guide, it's time to pause and reflect on the journey so far. This chapter will help you assess your progress, celebrate your achievements, and plan for the future as you continue on your path to lifelong wellness.

Section 1: Reflecting on Your Journey

Take some time to reflect on your health journey. Consider the progress you've made, the challenges you've overcome, and the habits you've established. Remember that every step, no matter how small, is a victory worth celebrating.

Section 2: Celebrating Your Achievements

Don't forget to celebrate your achievements. Whether it's reaching a fitness goal, sticking to a healthy eating plan, or simply feeling better in your everyday life, these milestones deserve recognition. Celebrating can also boost your motivation to continue on your wellness journey.

Section 3: Setting Future Goals

Now it's time to look ahead. What are your health and wellness goals for the future? These could be anything from running a marathon to mastering a complex yoga pose, or simply maintaining your current level of health. Remember, your goals should be realistic, attainable, and aligned with your values.

55

Section 4: Continuing Your Journey

Your health journey doesn't end here; it's a lifelong commitment. Keep learning, stay curious, and remain open to new experiences. Continue to adapt your wellness practices as your life changes, and always prioritize self-care.

In conclusion, reflecting on your journey, celebrating your achievements, setting future goals, and committing to continue are all crucial steps on your path to lifelong wellness. As we wrap up this guide, remember that health is a journey, not a destination. Stay committed, stay inspired, and enjoy the journey. You've got this!

Chapter 18

Embracing Balance: The Key to Lifelong Wellness

As you continue your journey towards lifelong health and wellness, it's crucial to remember the importance of balance. This final chapter will explore how to maintain a balanced approach to your health that encompasses physical activity, nutrition, mental well-being, and rest.

Section 1: Balancing Physical Activity and Rest

While regular physical activity is essential for good health, it's just as important to give your body time to rest and recover. Listen to your body and ensure you're incorporating rest days into your fitness routine.

Section 2: Nutritional Balance

Eating a balanced diet ensures your body gets the nutrients it needs. Rather than focusing on restriction, aim for a variety of foods from all food groups in appropriate proportions. Remember, it's okay to treat yourself occasionally!

Section 3: Mental and Emotional Balance

Your mental and emotional health are just as important as your physical health. Take time each day to do something you enjoy, practice mindfulness, and seek support when you need it.

Section 4: Work-Life Balance

Maintaining a healthy work-life balance can significantly impact your overall wellness. Make sure you're taking time for relaxation and recreation alongside your professional responsibilities.

In conclusion, balance is the key to sustaining your health and wellness journey in the long term. By balancing physical activity with rest, maintaining a balanced diet, prioritizing mental and emotional health, and ensuring a healthy work-life balance, you're setting yourself up for a lifetime of wellness. As we close this guide, remember - your health journey is unique to you. Stay true to yourself, stay committed, and keep moving forward. You're doing great!

Conclusion

Part 1: Reflecting on the Journey

As we draw this guide to a close, it's essential to take a moment to reflect on the journey we've embarked upon. We've navigated the realms of physical activity, nutrition, mental well-being, and the importance of balance in all aspects of health. We've recognized that wellness is not a destination, but a continuous journey that evolves with us through different stages of life.

Part 2: Acknowledging Achievements and Growth

Throughout this guide, you've taken steps towards understanding and implementing healthier habits. Whether you've made significant changes or small tweaks to your lifestyle, each step contributes to your overall wellness. Celebrate these achievements, no matter how small they may seem, as they signify personal growth and commitment to your health.

Part 3: Looking Forward to Lifelong Wellness

Finally, as we look ahead, remember that lifelong wellness is an ongoing commitment. It requires consistency, patience, and compassion towards oneself. Use what you've learned from this guide to continue shaping your unique wellness journey. Remember, there will be challenges along the way, but each one presents an opportunity for growth and learning. Keep striving for balance, prioritize self-care, and remain proactive in your pursuit of lifelong health. You are equipped with the knowledge and tools to make healthful choices and live a vibrant, fulfilling life.

I wish you success and Happiness in your journey,

Sincerely, Doctor AI

About the Author

Doctor AI is a distinguished author in the field of health and wellness, with an emphasis on empowering individuals to make informed decisions about their health. His work is distinguished by his ability to distill complex medical concepts into accessible, easy-to-understand language that puts the reader in control.

Dr. AI has always been at the forefront of integrating technological advancements into healthcare. His unique perspective combines an understanding of traditional medical principles with a forward-thinking approach to health tech.

His groundbreaking book, "Doctor AI, Longevity: The Long and the Short of It," revolutionized the way we view aging and longevity by providing readers with the latest research and developments in the field. This book provides actionable insights into how individuals can take control of their health and potentially extend their lifespan.

In his latest work, "Doctor AI, Weight Loss: What Have You Got to Lose?," Doctor AI turns his attention to one of the most pressing health issues facing society today - obesity and weight management. This book continues his mission of equipping readers with the knowledge they need to make informed decisions about their health. It covers the latest scientific findings on weight loss, diet, exercise, and the role of gut health, making it a must-read for anyone looking to achieve sustainable weight loss.

Doctor AI's books are more than just guides; they are tools designed to arm readers with professional facts, enabling them to take charge of their health. His work reflects his belief in the power of knowledge, empowering individuals to make healthier choices and live better lives.

With his keen insight, wealth of knowledge, and passion for empowering others, Doctor AI is truly a pioneer in the field of health and wellness literature. He continues to inspire readers worldwide to take control of their health journey.

Thanks for reading! Please add a short review on Amazon and let me know what you thought!

www.ingramcontent.com/pod-product-compliance
Lightning Source LLC
Chambersburg PA
CBHW060807260726

48660CB00002B/819